Copyright © 2021

All rights reserved. No part of this book may be reproduced in any form or by any electronic or mechanical means, including information storage and retrieval systems, without permission in writing from the publisher, except by reviewers, who may quote brief passages in a review

Table of Contents

30 Easy Ways to Lose Weight Naturally (Backed by Science)

There is a lot of bad weight loss information on the internet.

Much of what is recommended is questionable at best, and not based on any actual science.

However, there are several natural methods that have actually been proven to work.

Here are 30 easy ways to lose weight naturally.

1. Add Protein to Your Diet

When it comes to weight loss, protein is the king of nutrients.

Your body burns calories when digesting and metabolizing the protein you eat, so a high-protein diet can boost metabolism by up to 80–100 calories per day.

A high-protein diet can also make you feel more full and reduce your appetite. In fact, some studies show that people eat over 400 fewer calories per day on a high-protein diet.

Even something as simple as eating a high-protein breakfast (like eggs) can have a powerful effect.

2. Eat Whole, Single-Ingredient Foods

One of the best things you can do to become healthier is to base your diet on whole, single-ingredient foods.

By doing this, you eliminate the vast majority of added sugar, added fat and processed food.

Most whole foods are naturally very filling, making it a lot easier to keep within healthy calorie limits.

Furthermore, eating whole foods also provides your body with the many essential nutrients that it needs to function properly.

Weight loss often follows as a natural side effect of eating whole foods.

3. Avoid Processed Foods

Processed foods are usually high in added sugars, added fats and calories.

What's more, processed foods are engineered to make you eat as much as possible. They are much more likely to cause addictive-like eating than unprocessed foods.

4. Stock Up on Healthy Foods and Snacks

Studies have shown that the food you keep at home greatly affects weight and eating behavior.

By always having healthy food available, you reduce the chances of you or other family members eating unhealthy.

There are also many healthy and natural snacks that are easy to prepare and take with you on the go.

These include yogurt, whole fruit, nuts, carrots,and hard-boiled eggs.

5. Limit Your Intake of Added Sugar

Eating a lot of added sugar is linked with some of the world's leading diseases, including heart disease, type 2 diabetes and cancer.

On average, Americans eat about 15 teaspoons of added sugar each day. This amount is usually hidden in various processed foods, so you may be consuming a lot of sugar without even realizing it.

Since sugar goes by many names in ingredient lists, it can be very difficult to figure out how much sugar a product actually contains.

Minimizing your intake of added sugar is a great way to improve your diet.

6. Drink Water

There is actually truth to the claim that drinking water can help with weight loss.

Drinking 0.5 liters (17 oz) of water may increase the calories you burn by 24–30% for an hour afterward.

Drinking water before meals may also lead to reduced calorie intake, especially for middle-aged and older people.

Water is particularly good for weight loss when it replaces other beverages that are high in calories and sugar.

7. Drink (Unsweetened) Coffee

Fortunately, people are realizing that coffee is a healthy beverage that is loaded with antioxidants and other beneficial compounds.

Coffee drinking may support weight loss by increasing energy levels and the amount of calories you burn.

Caffeinated coffee may boost your metabolism by 3–11% and reduce your risk of developing type 2 diabetes by a whopping 23–50% .

Furthermore, black coffee is very weight loss friendly, since it can make you feel full but contains almost no calories.

8. Supplement With Glucomannan

Glucomannan is one of several weight loss pills that has been proven to work.

This water-soluble, natural dietary fiber comes from the roots of the konjac plant, also known as the elephant yam.

Glucomannan is low in calories, takes up space in the stomach and delays stomach emptying. It also reduces the absorption of protein and fat, and feeds the beneficial gut bacteria.

Its exceptional ability to absorb water is believed to be what makes it so effective for weight loss. One capsule is able to turn an entire glass of water into gel.

9. Avoid Liquid Calories

Liquid calories come from beverages like sugary soft drinks, fruit juices, chocolate milk and energy drinks.

These drinks are bad for health in several ways, including an increased risk of obesity. One study showed a drastic 60% increase in the risk of obesity among children, for each daily serving of a sugar-sweetened beverage.

It's also important to note that your brain does not register liquid calories the same way it does solid calories, so you end up adding these calories on top of everything else that you eat.

10. Limit Your Intake of Refined Carbs

Refined carbs are carbs that have had most of their beneficial nutrients and fiber removed.

The refining process leaves nothing but easily digested carbs, which can increase the risk of overeating and disease.

The main dietary sources of refined carbs are white flour, white bread, white rice, sodas, pastries, snacks, sweets, pasta, breakfast cereals, and added sugar.

11. Fast Intermittently

Intermittent fasting is an eating pattern that cycles between periods of fasting and eating.

There are a few different ways to do intermittent fasting, including the 5:2 diet, the 16:8 method and the eat-stop-eat method.

Generally, these methods make you eat fewer calories overall, without having to consciously restrict calories during the eating periods. This should lead to weight loss, as well as numerous other health benefits.

12. Drink (Unsweetened) Green Tea

Green tea is a natural beverage that is loaded with antioxidants.

Drinking green tea is linked with many benefits, such as increased fat burning and weight loss.

Green tea may increase energy expenditure by 4% and increase selective fat burning by up to 17%, especially harmful belly fat.

Matcha green tea is a variety of powdered green tea that may have even more powerful health benefits than regular green tea.

13. Eat More Fruits and Vegetables

Fruits and vegetables are extremely healthy, weight-loss-friendly foods.

In addition to being high in water, nutrients and fiber, they usually have very low energy density. This makes it possible to eat large servings without consuming too many calories.

Numerous studies have shown that people who eat more fruits and vegetables tend to weigh less.

14. Count Calories Once in a While

Being aware of what you're eating is very helpful when trying to lose weight.

There are several effective ways to do this, including counting calories, keeping a food diary or taking pictures of what you eat.

Using an app or another electronic tool may be even more beneficial than writing in a food diary.

15. Use Smaller Plates

Some studies have shown that using smaller plates helps you eat less, because it changes how you see portion sizes.

People seem to fill their plates the same, regardless of plate size, so they end up putting more food on larger plates than smaller ones.

Using smaller plates reduces how much food you eat, while giving you the perception of having eaten more.

16. Try a Low-Carb Diet

Many studies have shown that low-carb diets are very effective for weight loss.

Limiting carbs and eating more fat and protein reduces your appetite and helps you eat fewer calories.

This can result in weight loss that is up to 3 times greater than that from a standard low-fat diet.

A low-carb diet can also improve many risk factors for disease.

17. Eat More Slowly

If you eat too fast, you may eat way too many calories before your body even realizes that you are full.

Faster eaters are much more likely to become obese, compared to those who eat more slowly.

Chewing more slowly may help you eat fewer calories and increase the production of hormones that are linked to weight loss.

18. Replace Some Fat with Coconut Oil

Coconut oil is high in fats called medium-chain triglycerides, which are metabolized differently than other fats.

Studies show that they can boost your metabolism slightly, while helping you eat fewer calories.

Coconut oil may be especially helpful in reducing the harmful belly fat.

Note that this does not mean that you should add this fat to your diet, but simply replace some of your other fat sources with coconut oil.

19. Add Eggs to Your Diet

Eggs are the ultimate weight loss food. They are cheap, low in calories, high in protein and loaded with all sorts of nutrients.

High-protein foods have been shown to reduce appetite and increase fullness, compared to foods that contain less protein.

Furthermore, eating eggs for breakfast may cause up to 65% greater weight loss over 8 weeks, compared to eating bagels for breakfast. It may also help you eat fewer calories throughout the rest of the day.

20. Spice Up Your Meals

Chili peppers and jalapenos contain a compound called capsaicin, which may boost metabolism and increase the burning of fat.

Capsaicin may also reduce appetite and calorie intake.

21. Take Probiotics

Probiotics are live bacteria that have health benefits when eaten. They can improve digestive health and heart health, and may even help with with weight loss.

Studies have shown that overweight and obese people tend to have different gut bacteria than normal-weight people, which may influence weight.

Probiotics may help regulate the healthy gut bacteria. They may also block the absorption of dietary fat, while reducing appetite and inflammation.

Of all the probiotic bacteria, Lactobacillus gasseri shows the most promising effects on weight loss.

22. Get Enough Sleep

Getting enough sleep is incredibly important for weight loss, as well as to prevent future weight gain.

Studies have shown that sleep-deprived people are up to 55% more likely to become obese, compared to those who get enough sleep. This number is even higher for children.

This is partly because sleep deprivation disrupts the daily

fluctuations in appetite hormones, leading to poor appetite regulation.

23. Eat More Fiber

Fiber-rich foods may help with weight loss.

Foods that contain water-soluble fiber may be especially helpful, since this type of fiber can help increase the feeling of fullness.

Fiber may delay stomach emptying, make the stomach expand and promote the release of satiety hormones.

Ultimately, this makes us eat less naturally, without having to think about it.

Furthermore, many types of fiber can feed the friendly gut bacteria. Healthy gut bacteria have been linked with a reduced risk of obesity.

Just make sure to increase your fiber intake gradually to avoid abdominal discomfort, such as bloating, cramps and diarrhea.

24. Brush Your Teeth After Meals

Many people brush or floss their teeth after eating, which may help limit the desire to snack or eat between meals.

This is because many people do not feel like eating after brushing their teeth. Plus, it can make food taste bad.

Therefore, if you brush or use mouthwash after eating, you may be be less tempted to grab an unnecessary snack.

25. Combat Your Food Addiction

Food addiction involves overpowering cravings and changes in your brain chemistry that make it harder to resist eating certain foods.

This is a major cause of overeating for many people, and affects a significant percentage of the population. In fact, a recent 2014 study found that almost 20% of people fulfilled the criteria for food addiction.

Some foods are much more likely to cause symptoms of addiction than others. This includes highly processed junk foods that are high in sugar, fat or both.

The best way to beat food addiction is to seek help.

26. Do Some Sort of Cardio

Doing cardio — whether it is jogging, running, cycling, power walking or hiking — is a great way to burn calories and improve both mental and physical health.

Cardio has been shown to improve many risk factors for heart disease. It can also help reduce body weight.

Cardio seems to be particularly effective at reducing the dangerous belly fat that builds up around your organs and causes metabolic disease.

27. Add Resistance Exercises

Loss of muscle mass is a common side effect of dieting.

If you lose a lot of muscle, your body will start burning fewer calories than before.

By lifting weights regularly, you'll be able to prevent this loss in muscle mass.

As an added benefit, you'll also look and feel much better.

28. Use Whey Protein

Most people get enough protein from diet alone. However, for those who don't, taking a whey protein supplement is an effective way to boost protein intake.

One study shows that replacing part of your calories with whey protein can cause significant weight loss, while also increasing lean muscle mass.

Just make sure to read the ingredients list, because some varieties are loaded with added sugar and other unhealthy additives.

29. Practice Mindful Eating

Mindful eating is a method used to increase awareness while eating.

It helps you make conscious food choices and develop awareness of your hunger and satiety cues. It then helps you eat healthy in response to those cues.

Mindful eating has been shown to have significant effects on weight, eating behavior and stress in obese individuals. It is especially helpful against binge eating and emotional eating.

By making conscious food choices, increasing your awareness and listening to your body, weight loss should follow naturally and easily.

30. Focus on Changing Your Lifestyle

Dieting is one of those things that almost always fails in the long term. In fact, people who "diet" tend to gain more weight over time.

Instead of focusing only on losing weight, make it a primary goal to nourish your body with healthy food and nutrients.

Eat to become a healthier, happier, fitter person — not just to lose weight.

Are Protein Shakes Good For Weight Loss

Weight gain and obesity are increasingly becoming a health risk to individuals in recent years, and the notion that those problems are caused by lack of willpower doesn't do any justice. Although weight gain is largely a product of eating behavior and lifestyle, some individuals are not entirely in control of their body size. Overweight and obesity can be caused by several factors, including genetics and hormones, making some people predisposed to gaining weight. Many turn to weight loss interventions such as workouts and protein shakes. So, are protein shakes good for weight loss?

Despite the predisposition to gain weight, people can overcome their genetic disadvantages by changing their lifestyle and behavior. It is not a simple task, but it can be accomplished through willpower, dedication, and perseverance. One of the most popular strategies for weight loss is to follow a high protein diet because protein curbs one's appetite, thus resulting in the reduction of the total calories consumed in a day.

What Are Protein Shakes?

Due to the importance they play or are perceived to play, the world of protein shakes is vast and does not seem to end. They come in different types, flavors, and formulations for any conceivable dietary need under the sun. Based on your preference, you can purchase premixed, ready-to-drink bottles, or protein powder.

The conception behind protein shakes is that they are meal replacements meant to help people lose weight. Because protein is filling, it may aid in suppressing your appetite by keeping in check your hunger hormones.

Most protein shakes for weight loss work by having a person replace either one or two meals per day with a shake, and then the third meal should be small and with low calories. In some extreme protein shakes diets, one drinks the shakes only for several days without any other food, but most professionals disapprove of this method.

The protein shakes can prove to be a valuable weight loss tool when consumed moderately. To be truly effective and healthy, they need to be paired with a couple of other sustainable lifestyle changes.

How Does The Protein Shake Diet Work?

To begin with, protein shakes offer more than just protein. Many manufacturers tend to fortify the shakes with a variety of vitamins and other minerals. Some may even have fruits, vegetables, and other essential nutrients. The important question here is, why are protein shakes good for weight loss?

A link has been established between the consumption of proteins and an increased feeling of fullness. It, therefore, follows that people who include enough protein in their daily diets ought to have fewer food cravings, and hence they will eat less. Some choose to get the protein through shakes. Below is a sample of a protein diet daily meal plan:

- Two protein shakes (between 200 and 300 calories each)

- Three small snacks (about 100 calories each)

- One full meal such as dinner (between 400 and 500 calories)

Based on this diet plan, the protein shakes are to be taken in the morning and at lunchtime. This is a very low calorie meal plan which should always be discussed with and monitored by a physician.

Are protein shakes for breakfast good for weight loss? There cannot be protein shakes as effective as the breakfast ones. This is because when you wake up, it is when you are hungry the most and will be tempted to eat a lot. Substituting your normal heavy breakfast with protein shakes already reduces the amount of food you eat. Most importantly, the protein shake will keep you feeling full. Hence you won't be craving more food.

When To Have Protein Shakes?

Another good time to consume a protein shake is after a workout. This is the point at which your body needs instant nourishment for muscle recovery and growth. The recommended consumption window is 30 to 45 minutes after your workout. This timeline is important because protein uptake is usually faster after a workout. You can also take the shake 30 minutes before your workout to energize yourself and boost your stamina.

How Good Are Protein Shakes for Weight Loss?

Are high protein shakes good for weight loss? When taken properly, protein shakes can be very effective in weight loss and control. That said, you must be aware that protein shakes alone are not the magic bullet for your body goals. Incorporate an overall healthy diet and a workout plan, and you will be amazed by the results. Below are some of the benefits of protein shakes to weight loss:

- Weight loss: Don't forget that the reason why you are drinking protein shakes in the first place is to lose weight. Getting enough protein is crucial in the weight loss journey and weight maintenance. Protein shakes achieve weight loss in several ways, including the fact that protein is more filling than carbs.

- Appetite control: Even people who are not keen on losing weight but have appetite problems can benefit from protein shakes. Protein is good for controlling appetite because it is dense and takes longer to digest. This means that you will remain full for much longer and wouldn't eat in that period. Protein also controls appetite by regulating ghrelin, which is the hunger hormone.

• Stable blood sugar levels: Protein can help stabilize your blood sugar levels. Sometimes blood sugar dips between meals, but it can be kept in check by the inclusion of a bit more protein in your meals.

• Building muscle: Intake of strategic supplementation with a protein, such as whey, can be good for muscle growth. Muscle growth is accelerated even more when you pair the protein with a resistance exercise. This will help your body to be leaner and have more stability (4).

- Metabolism: Protein works to increase the thermic effect of food. The thermic effect of food relates to the number of calories you burn by digesting what you eat. With an increased metabolism rate, your chances of losing weight are very high.

Risks And Side Effects

• Meal replacement shakes should not completely replace a healthy, balanced diet. Doing so could be harmful because there is no way you can get all the essential nutrients from just a single food source. You may end up losing more weight than you anticipated or even leave your body vulnerable to diseases.

• If the body does not get enough calories and nutrients, there is the risk that you might experience problems with metabolism. The result will be slowing or disrupting your weight loss plan. Furthermore, eating a varied diet reduces your chances of having obesity.

• A good number of protein shakes utilize large sweetener quantities to improve their flavor, and this can trigger blood sugar spikes.

• Consuming too much protein over the long term may not be good for your body. It may cause you problems in the kidneys and bones and even increase the risk of certain cancers.

- Some protein shakes contain unsafe levels of contaminants such as mercury, arsenic, lead, and cadmium. These contaminants can potentially cause serious health problems, some of which are life-threatening.

- Because they are nutritional supplements, protein shakes are not subject to stringent regulations, as is the case with medicine, and marketing materials of these products may sometimes be misleading.

Types Of Protein

There is no limit to the number of different protein options available in the market, so you have to figure one which is right for you. If you are lucky, you might find one that matches your Myers-Briggs personality type.

What protein shakes are good for weight loss? Here are some:

Whey

Whey is undoubtedly one of the most, if not the most, common and inexpensive type of protein. The protein is isolated from cow's milk and is readily absorbed. It is very efficient in building muscle, and the good thing about it is its availability. You can easily get it off any counter just in case you are experiencing a protein emergency.

Are whey protein shakes good for weight loss? Whey protein does not only help you gain muscle but also lose fat as well. However, it must be combined with exercise to see weight loss results.

Casein

This type of protein is also isolated from the milk of a cow, but it is not as effective in building muscle as whey. One other disadvantage is that it is a bit more expensive. Casein takes longer than whey to digest. This means it will keep you feeling full for a longer period, which is especially a good thing when you are trying to lose weight.

Egg

The egg-based protein powder is a good solid option for the liquid shake.

This type of protein has the upper hand because it is very easy for your body to absorb. The downside is that it is only made with the egg whites, hence, the consumers will be missing out on the many benefits of the yolk.

Soy

The good thing with protein shakes is that they accommodate even individuals who have gone vegan. Soy protein is among the best when it comes to plant-based diets because it is a complete protein. This means that soy protein contains all the essential amino acids that your body requires, just like with animal proteins.

There is a controversy surrounding soy because it has phytoestrogens, which allegedly have effects on hormones, although the overall body of scientific evidence suggests that soy is perfectly safe to consume.

Pea

Pea may be the subject of many juvenile jokes, but its protein is as good as any other plant-based protein. It is an alternative solid choice, especially for vegetarians. Although it is a complete protein, it is a little low in the amino acid methionine. Good thing that this can be quickly remedied by adding nut butter or nut milk to your pea protein shake, and you are good to go.

Hemp

As is the case with soy and pea, hemp is also a plant-based protein. It is also a complete protein. Another advantage of hemp is that it is a good source of healthy omega-3 fats. Its amino acid lysine content is slightly lower, a situation that can be rectified by adding tofu or almond butter to the hemp protein shake, or simply varying your plant protein sources from shake to shake or meal to meal.

Rice

Brown rice protein powder is one of the most common vegan protein choices. It is relatively cheap and happens to be a complete protein. It is similar to hemp due to its low lysine.

Homemade Protein Shakes For Weight Loss

Why buy protein shakes when you can make them at home? Sometimes you may not trust the protein shakes that are made in a factory, or you may not have the money to buy the shakes day after day. Worry not because there are several homemade protein shakes you can try.

But, are pure protein shakes good for weight loss? There are many benefits other than weight loss to be expected from the homemade protein shakes below:

Peanut butter protein shake

The homemade peanut butter protein shake gives you a nutty, creamy, and delicious feel. The upside with this shake is that it does not contain added sugar, and it is high in fiber and low in fat. Prepare it by blending 1 cup of yogurt, ½ cup of almond milk, 1 to 2 tablespoons of peanut butter, and 15-20 green grapes. Refrigerate the mixture and enjoy it chilled.

Chocolate and a banana protein shake

Chocolate! Are chocolate protein shakes good for weight loss? It may be unheard of, but chocolate and bananas do make a great combination and are also very good for weight loss. In addition to having great taste, they also make your protein shake super healthy. To prepare it, you need 10 almonds, ½ cup of yogurt, ¾ cup of milk, ½ teaspoon cinnamon, ¼ cup of cooked quinoa, 1 banana cut into chunks, and 1 tablespoon of cocoa powder. Blend the mixture in the blender.

Berry protein shake

All types of berries are efficient antioxidants and twice as a great source of fiber, which is important in your weight loss journey. You can opt to use strawberries, blackberries, or even gooseberries in your smoothie. The recipe includes 7-10 berries, ½ cup of whipped cottage cheese, ¼ cup of water, 1 tablespoon of chia seeds, and a little honey, but it is optional.

Vegan protein shake

Is plant-based protein shakes good for you for weight loss? Most plant-based protein shakes are complete proteins that make them a great alternative for individuals keen on losing some pounds. The vegan protein shake is designed for individuals who decided to stop the consumption of milk and dairy products but are still in need of a high protein shake for weight loss.

To make the vegan protein shake blend, you need ¾ cup of silken tofu, 1 cup of almond or cashew milk, 1 banana, ¼ cup of cooked oats, 1 teaspoon of honey (or agave or other syrup), and 1 teaspoon of vanilla essence for flavor.

Raw egg protein shake

The raw egg protein shake is not only important for weight loss but also muscle building. The main ingredient of the homemade protein shake is raw egg, and you must ensure that the eggs you use are of good quality. The shake is made by mixing 1 raw egg including its yolk, ½ avocado, ½ cup of milk or coconut milk, 1 banana, 1 teaspoon of honey, and ½ teaspoon of cinnamon. To prepare, place all the ingredients in a blender and blend them.

Spinach flax protein shake

It is a green homemade shake prepared by combining 1 cup of unsweetened almond milk or any other kind of milk, spinach leaves, ½ cup of mango chunks, ½ cup of pineapple bits, ½ banana, 1 tablespoon of flax seeds, and 1 tablespoon of chia seeds. Blend the mixture and serve immediately.

Important Considerations

• Before you commence on a protein shake diet, reflect on whether you can manage your daily schedule if you eat just one meal per day. Remember that a protein shake isn't a meal but merely a meal replacement. Your body system may go into shock from eating three meals per day to drinking two of them. Another option would be to consume a normal 3-meal per day diet and include protein shakes as pre- or post-workout snacks.

- Also, take into consideration the duration you can or should use shakes as meal replacements. A moderate diet will enable you to lose about 1 to 2 pounds per week. This will determine the period in which you keep the diet going based on the number of pounds you intend to lose. Losing weight more quickly than this is not healthy or sustainable, so make sure you are consuming enough calories every day to nourish and fuel your body.

- The diet can only be successful if the snacks you incorporate and the daily meal(s) are nutritious and healthy.

You do not want your body to become weak due to poor dietary choices. It goes without saying that if the snacks or meals are not nutritious, then the results will not be as desired.

• Even though you will be on protein shakes, you will have to continue shopping for some groceries. That aside, you must establish that you have the willpower to stick to the diet plan. After taking the shake, you will probably feel that you haven't eaten what you are used to eating.

- You will need a lot of courage to avoid other unhealthy snack foods, especially if your workplace or home environment is filled with those foods. It won't make any sense to drink protein shakes once or twice a day and then overeat the rest of the time.

The Bottom Line

Are protein shakes good for weight loss? Many people have been in a place where they wondered if the before-and-after photos on some of the protein shake ads are legit. One of the reasons why protein shakes are very popular is because they are super convenient, and all one has to do is drink them. The good thing is that there is a lot of information available on how to use them efficiently. However, even though protein shakes have some benefits that may result in weight loss, they alone cannot guarantee weight loss.

Diets are great, but your body will thank you if you supplement your healthy nutrition plan with a good workout. Take up this 20 Min Full Body Workout at Home.